I0428315

The Quick and Clean Detox: Easy Recipes That Flush Your Body of Harmful Toxins and Kill Cravings

Disclaimer and Terms of Use: Effort has been made to ensure that the information in this book is accurate and complete, however, the author and the publisher do not warrant the accuracy of the information, text and graphics contained within the book due to the rapidly changing nature of science, research, known and unknown facts and internet. The Author and the publisher do not hold any responsibility for errors, omissions or contrary interpretation of the subject matter herein. This book is presented solely for motivational and informational purposes only.

Table of Contents

Berry Detox

Ingredients:

- 1 C frozen raspberries
- ¾ C almond milk
- ¼ C cherries, pitted
- 1 ½ T honey
- 2 tsp fresh ginger
- 1 tsp flaxseed
- 1 tsp. lemon juice

Directions: Blend and serve

Green

Ingredients:

- 1 ¼ C kale leaves
- 1 ¼ C cubed mango
- 2 celery ribs, chopped
- 1 C orange juice
- ¼ C leaf parsley, chopped
- ¼ C fresh mint, chopped

Directions:

I.   Blend and serve

Hale Kale

Ingredients:

- ½ pear
- ¼ avocado
- ½ Cucumber
- ½ lemon
- Cilantro
- 1 C Kale
- 1" ginger
- 1 S protein powder
- Water

Directions:

I.   Blend and serve

Blue Spirit

Ingredients:

- ½ banana
- ½ C blueberries
- ¼ avocado
- ½ C almond milk
- 1 tsp Spirulina
- 1 S Vanilla protein powder
- Water

Directions:

I.   Blend and Serve

Alkaline Detox

Ingredients:

- ½ pear
- ¼ avocado
- 1 C spinach
- ¼ C coconut water
- 1 C almond milk
- 1 tsp chia seeds
- 1 S protein powder
- Water

Directions:

I.   Blend and serve

Belly Detox

Ingredients

- 1 C papaya
- 1 C coconut kefir
- ½ lime, juice
- 1 T raw honey

Directions

I.   Blend and serve

Smooth Detox

Ingredients:

- 5 lettuce leaves
- ½ granny apple
- ¼ avocado
- ½ cucumber
- ½ C jicama
- Cilantro
- 1 lime
- 4 S hemp protein
- Water

Directions

I. Blend and Serve

Morning Glory Detox

Ingredients:

- 1 cucumber
- 1 C kale
- 1 C romaine
- Celery, chopped
- 1 green apple, cored
- 1 broccoli stemmed
- ½ lemon, peeled

Directions:

I.   Blend and serve

Goddess Detox

Ingredients:

- 1avocado
- 1banana
- 1 C blueberries
- 1 cucumber
- Spinach
- Coconut water

Directions:

I.   Blend and serve

Red Berry detox

Ingredients:

- 3 C cashews
- 2 C strawberries, stemmed
- 1 orange, peeled
- 1 banana
- 1 ½ C spinach

Directions:

I.   Blend and serve

Italian Detox

Ingredients:

- 6 carrots
- 2-3 tomatoes
- 1-2 red bell peppers
- 4 T minced garlic
- Celery, chopped
- 1 C watercress
- 1 C spinach
- 1 jalapeno, seeded

Directions:

I.   Blend and Serve

Berry Detox

Ingredients:

- 1 C alkaline water
- ¼ C blueberries
- 1 lemon

Directions:

I.   Blend and Serve

Goji Detox

Ingredients:

- 1 C coconut Kefir
- 1 banana (frozen)
- ¼ C frozen strawberries
- 3 T goji

Directions:

I. Blend and Serve

Ginger Milk Detox

Ingredients:

- 1 C almond milk
- ½ C blueberries
- 1 banana
- 3 T ginger

Directions:

I.   Blend and Serve

Mint berry

Ingredients:

- ½ green apple
- 2 T hemp hearts
- Mint leaves
- Green leaves
- ¼ C frozen berry blend
- 12 oz. water

Directions:

I.   Blend and Serve

Sensual Detox (See our book of Bedroom Smoothies)

Ingredients:

- 1 T cacao powder
- 2 T hemp seeds
- 4 ½ endive leaves
- Stevia pkt
- 12 oz. water

Directions:

I.   Blend and Serve

Green Power Detox

Ingredients:

- 1 green apple, cored
- 1 lemon, whole
- 1 tsp barley juice (grass juice)
- 1 cucumber, peeled
- Red lettuce leaves
- ¼ C frozen mango
- 10 oz. water

Directions:

I.   Blend and Serve

Liver Cleanser

Ingredients:

- ¼ C Parsley
- 1 small beet, wedged
- 1 apple, cored and seeded
- 1 peeled lemon
- ½" ginger root
- 1 T chia seeds
- Water

Directions:

I.   Blend and Serve

Glowing Skin Detox

Ingredients:

- ½ cucumber
- 1pear, cored and seeded
- 1 lemon, peeled
- 1 orange, peeled
- 1 T pumpkin seeds
- Water

Directions:

I.   Blend and Serve

Detox Tonic

Ingredients:

- 1 C almond milk
- 1 ½ T maca powder
- 2 T chia seeds
- 1 S vanilla protein powder
- 1 ripe banana
- 1 Stevia pkt
- 1 ½ T cacao nibs

Directions:

I.   Blend and serve

Clear Skin detox

Ingredients:

- 1 C coconut Kefir
- ½ C parsley
- 1 cucumber, seeded
- 1 apple
- 1 T coconut oil
- 1 lime
- 2 T mint leaves

Directions:

I.   Blend and Serve

Elixir Detox

Ingredients:

- 1 C almond milk
- 1 C blueberries
- ½ C raspberries
- 2 T goji berries, soaked
- 1 T coconut oil
- 1 T flaxseed
- 2 dates, soaked

Directions:

I.   Blend and Serve

Youth Detox Smoothie

Ingredients:

- 1 C almond milk
- ½ C Kale
- Spinach
- ½ C cilantro
- Green apples, cored
- 1 T green algae

Directions:

I.   Blend and serve

Cranberry Detox

Ingredients:

- ½ C cranberries
- 1 celery stalks, chopped
- 1 cucumber
- 1 apple, cored
- 1 pear, cored
- Spinach

Directions:

I.   Blend and Serve

Fat Flush

Ingredients:

- 1 red beet
- 2 carrots
- 1 radish
- 2 T minced garlic
- Parsley

Directions:

I.   Blend and serve

www.ingramcontent.com/pod-product-compliance
Lightning Source LLC
Chambersburg PA
CBHW070941290526
45795CB00003B/1107